Paleo

CW00523414

The Complete Book of Paleo Diet ,Natural Way to Lose
Weight And Get A Healthy Body

(All You Need To Know About The Paleo Diet)

Domingo Poole

TABLE OF CONTENTS

Spice Infused Mashed Potatoes

Ingredients:

1/2 tsp Cumin seed powder

2 cup Curd

2 tsp Honey

Salt to taste

2 tbsp fresh Coriander leaves

2 medium sized Potatoes

1/2 tsp green Chili paste

1/2 tsp Clove powder

1/2 tsp Cinnamon powder

Instructions:

1. Cook the potatoes in boiling water.

2. Once they are boiled, remove the skin and mash the potatoes to a thick paste.

3. Add the chili paste, clove powder, cinnamon powder, cumin seed powder, curd and honey to the mashed potatoes.

4. Add salt and mix well, garnish with fresh coriander leaves before serving.

Potatoes In Green Lemon Chutney

Ingredients:

1/2 tsp Coriander seed powder

1/2 tsp Cumin seeds

1/2 tsp Asafetida

2 tsp grated coconut pulp

2 medium sized Potatoes

1/2 tsp green Chili paste

4 tbsp fresh Coriander leaves

2 tsp fresh Lemon juice

3-4 tbsp Cooking Oil

Salt to taste

Instructions:

1. Make holes in the potatoes with a fork and then boil them in water.
2. Once the potatoes are cooked, peel off the skin and cut them into small bite size pieces.
3. Making *Green Lemon Chutney* –
4. Grind chili paste and coriander leaves into a thick paste.
5. Add lemon juice and coriander seed powder to the paste. This is the green lemon chutney.
6. Mix the green lemon chutney, salt and potatoes in a bowl and stir well.
7. Heat the cooking oil in a pan.
8. Once the oil is hot, add the cumin seeds and asafetida.
9. When cumin starts to crackle, turn off the heat and add the contents of the pan to the chutney coated potatoes in the bowl.

10. Mix well and garnish with grated coconut pulp.

Green Potato Kebab

Ingredients:

2 cup Cottage Cheese

2 cup fresh Coriander leaves

2 tsp Ginger-Garlic paste

1/2 tsp Coriander seed powder

2-4 medium sized Potatoes

2 cups fresh Green Peas

1 tsp green Chilly paste

2 cups fresh Spinach leaves

Salt to taste

4-6 tbsp Cooking Oil

Instructions:

1. Boil the Potatoes and green peas.

2. Remove the skin of the potatoes and mash them into a thick paste.

3. Also mash the peas into a paste and mix it thoroughly with the mashed potatoes.

4. Finely chop the spinach leaves, mix them with grated cottage cheese. Once thoroughly mixed add the chili paste, chopped coriander leaves, coriander seed powder and ginger-garlic paste.

5. Then add this green kebab mixture to the potato-green pea paste. Once mixed thoroughly make small balls of this mixture.

6. Heat the cooking oil in a pan.

7. Once the oil is hot, put the green kebab balls into the pan and shallow fry them, serve hot.

8. (the green kebab's taste   when dipped in curd or eaten with a bite of tomato salsa)

Crispy Sour Plantains

Ingredients:

2 tbsp Tamarind pulp

4 -4 tbsp Cooking Oil

Salt to taste

2 plantains

1/2 tsp red Chili powder

2 cup Rice flour

Instructions:

1. Remove the skin of the plantains and slice them into thin wheels.
2. Rub salt, red chili powder and tamarind pulp to these slices thoroughly and leave the slices to marinate for 4 0-40 min.
3. Heat the cooking oil in a pan.

4. Once the oil is hot, shallow fry the slices Fry till crispy. Garnish with fresh coriander leaves and serve hot.

Carrot Chutney

Ingredients:

1/2 tsp Cumin seeds

1/2 tsp red Chili powder

1/2 tsp Sugar

3-4 tbsp Cooking Oil

240 gm fresh Carrots

4 tbsp Sesame seeds

1 cup of grated Coconut pulp (dried)

4 tbsp roughly grated Almonds

2-4 Curry leaves

1/2 tsp Asafetida

1/2 tsp Mustard seeds

1/2 tsp Turmeric powder

Instructions:

1. Finely grate the carrots, then spread them over a flat tray and sun-dry them for a few hours till the moisture dries up.
2. Heat the cooking oil in a pan.
3. Once the oil is hot, add the cumin seeds, asafetida, mustard seeds and turmeric powder.
4. Once the cumin starts crackling, add the curry leaves followed by the dried grated carrots, sesame seeds and grated almonds.

5. Stir for a minute and then add grated coconut pulp, red chili powder, sugar and salt.
6. Don't cover the pan and stir the carrots till they become crispy.

Crunchy-Sour Cucumber

Ingredients:

2 tbsp fresh Coriander leaves

2-4 tsp fresh lemon juice

1/2 tsp Sugar

1/2 tsp Cumin seeds

2-4 tbsp Cooking Oil

Salt to taste

220 gm fresh Cucumbers

4 tbsp roughly grated Almonds

1/2 tsp green Chili powder

2 tbsp grated Coconut pulp

Instructions:

1. Peel off the skin of the cucumbers and finely slice them into thin slices.
2. Put these slices in a bowl.
3. Heat the cooking oil in a pan.
4. Once the oil is hot, add the cumin seeds and green chili paste, stir for a minute and then pour the contents of the pan over the cucumber slices.
5. Then add grated coconut pulp, chopped coriander leaves, sugar and salt to the cucumber slices and stir well.
6. Then add the lemon juice to the cucumber, stir a bit and serve fresh.

Instant Cucumber Pickle

Ingredients:

1/2 tsp Turmeric powder

1/2 tsp red Chili powder

2 tbsp Coriander leaves (finely chopped)

2 tsp Salt

3-4 tbsp Cooking Oil

240 gm fresh Cucumber

2 tsp Mustard seeds

1 tsp Fenugreek seeds

3-4 tsp Lemon juice

1/2 tsp Asafetida

Instructions:

1. Peel off the skin of the cucumbers and finely dice them in small bite sized pieces. Remove them in a bowl.
2. Then sprinkle turmeric powder, red chili powder and salt over the cucumbers and leave it for 8-25 minutes.
3. You will notice that cucumber secrets fair amount of water. Remove this water in a cup.
4. Do not throw this water away. Grind 1 tsp of fenugreek seeds and 1 tsp of mustard seed in this water into a paste.
5. Rub this paste evenly to the diced cucumbers and also add the lemon juice to the diced cucumbers.
6. Heat the cooking oil in a pan.
7. Once the oil is hot, add the remaining mustard seeds and asafetida to the pan and stir for a minute. When mustard seeds

crackle, add the contents of the pan to the cucumbers and mix well.

8. Garnish with coriander leaves and serve fresh.

Coconut-Bengal Gram Chutney

Ingredients:

1 tsp green Chili paste

1 cup fresh Curd

1/2 tsp Mustard seeds

1/2 tsp Asafetida

3-4 tbsp Cooking Oil

2 cup fresh grated Coconut pulp

2 tbsp split Bengal Grams

2 tbsp split Black Grams

2 Curry leaves

Salt to taste

Instructions:

1. Soak bengal grams and black grams for at least 2-2 ½ hrs, then keep them on a strainer to let all water drain off.
2. Heat the cooking oil in a pan.
3. Once the oil is hot, add the mustard seeds, curry leaves and asafetida to the pan.
4. When the mustard seeds start to crackle add the bengal gram and black gram to the pan, stir it for a while and then cover the pan with a lid and let it cook for 8 -8 minutes.
5. Once it is cooked, remove the lid and add the green chili paste, stir for a few seconds and then put the

lid back on and cook for minute or
so.

6. Then remove the lid and add the
grated coconut pulp to the pan and
mix it all well, stir for a minute
more and then turn-off the heat.

7. Once it cools down, add the curd
and salt to it, mix thoroughly and
serve with a garnish of chopped
fresh coriander leaves.

Green Mango Chutney

Ingredients:

1/2 tsp green Chili paste

2 1 tbsp fresh Coriander leaves (finely chopped)

1 tbsp Olive Oil

Salt to taste

2 medium sized raw green mangoes

4 tbsp grated Coconut pulp

Instructions:

1. Finely grate the raw mangoes.
2. Then add the grated coconut pulp and green chili paste to the grated mangoes and mix it well.

3. Then add the olive oil and mix again.
4. Then add the salt to this mixture and mix again.
5. You'll notice that a lot of water is secreted by the mangoes, when you add salt. (don't remove this water)

Potato Chutney

Ingredients:

2 tbsp fresh Coriander leaves (chopped)

1/2 tsp asafetida

1/2 tsp Turmeric powder

2 medium sized Potato

1/2 tsp green Chili paste

4 tbsp grated Coconut pulp

Instructions:

1. Boil the potato for a few minutes in water. (don't cook it completely, just let it remain in boiling water for some time.)
2. Then peel off its skin and finely grate it.

3. Add green chili paste, grated coconut, chopped coriander leaves and salt to the potatoes and mix well.
4. Then add asafetida and turmeric powder to this mixture and grind it into a thick coarse paste.

Ripe Mango in Sour Sauce

Ingredients:

1/2 tsp Mustard seeds

2 tsp Tamarind Pulp

1/2 tsp Sugar

Salt

2 medium size Ripe Mango

1 cup fresh grated Coconut pulp

1/2 tsp red Chili powder

Instructions:

1. Remove the skin of the mango and cut it into small pieces.
2. Grind grated coconut pulp, mustard seeds, red chili powder and salt into a thick paste. (add 2-4 tsp water while grinding)

3. Add the mango to this paste and mix well.
4. Then add the tamarind pulp and sugar finally. Stir well till sugar dissolves.
5. Serve while fresh.

Spicy Pineapple Stew

Ingredients:

1 tsp Cumin seeds

1/2 tsp Mustard seeds

1/2 tsp Turmeric powder

3-4 tbsp Cooking Oil

2 Curry Leaves

2 1 cup ripe Pineapple (finely diced)

2 tbsp grated Jaggery

1/2 tsp red Chili powder

2 cup grated Coconut pulp

Salt to taste

Instructions:

1. Grind grated coconut pulp, 1/2 tsp cumin seeds, 1/2 tsp mustard seeds together into a thick paste.
2. Add 2 cup of water to a pan and bring it to a boil, then add the diced pineapple, turmeric powder, red chili powder and salt to the water and let it cook for 4-10 minutes.
3. Then add jaggery to it and stir till it dissolves and then add the paste we have made earlier and mix well. This is the stew base.
4. Heat the cooking oil in another pan.
5. Once the oil is hot, add the cumin seeds, curry leaves.
6. Once the cumin starts crackling, pour the contents of the pan to the stew base and stir for a bit and then turn off the heat under the stew.
7. The Pineapple stew is ready, serve hot.

Stirred Cabbage With Black Gram

Ingredients:

1 tsp Asafetida

1 tsp Mustard seeds

2-4 Curry leaves

 Salt to taste

2 medium sized Cabbage

2 tbsp split Black Gram

2 dried red chili

3-4 tbsp Cooking Oil

Instructions:

1. Soak the split Black Gram overnight. (must be soaked for a minimum 6 hrs.)
2. Clean the Cabbage and chop it finely into thin strips.
3. Heat the cooking oil in a pan.
4. Once the oil is hot, add Curry leaves, Mustard seeds, asafetida and the dried chili.
5. Once the Mustard seeds start crackling, add the split Black Gram.
6. Lower the flame and stir the contents in the pan for a couple of minutes.
7. Then add the chopped Cabbage to the pan, add salt to taste and cover the pan with a lid and serve hot once the cabbage is cooked.

Curd Cooked Bitter Gourd

Ingredients:

1/2 tsp red Chili powder

2 tsp Turmeric powder

1/2 tsp Cumin seeds

1/2 tsp Mustard seeds

1/2 tsp Asafetida

3-4 tbsp Cooking Oil

2 cups of Curd

220 gm Bitter Gourd

1/2 tsp Coriander seed powder

Instructions:

Cut and clean the bitter gourd.

Wash it with water and then grate the bitter gourd.

Add turmeric and salt to the bitter gourd; mix it well and leave for 2 hr.

After an hour squeeze out all the water from the bitter gourd.

Heat the cooking oil in a pan.

Once the oil is hot, add the cumin seeds, mustard seeds, asafetida and chili powder.

After the mustard seeds start crackling add the bitter gourd to the pan.

Stir well and cover up with a lid and let it cook over its own steam.

After a few minutes add the curd and coriander seed powder to the pan

Keep stirring the contents of the pan continuously till the bitter gourd is completely cooked.

Serve while hot.

Flour Infused Snake Gourd

Ingredients:

1/2 tsp red Chili powder

1/2 tsp Turmeric powder

1/2 tsp Cumin seeds

1/2 tsp Mustard seeds

1/2 tsp Asafetida

2-4 tbsp Cooking Oil

280 gm fresh Snake Gourd

2 medium Onion

1 cup Chickpea flour

1/2 tsp Coriander seed powder

Instructions:

1. Peel off the skin of the snake gourd, remove the seeds and dice it finely and then clean it with water.
2. Finely dice the onion.
3. Heat the cooking oil in a pan.
4. Once the oil is hot, add the cumin seeds, mustard seeds, asafetida and chili powder.
5. Once the mustard starts crackling, add the diced fresh onion and stir till it becomes pink.
6. Add the snake gourd, stir for 2 minutes then add the coriander seed powder and Turmeric powder.
7. Add salt to taste, and place a lid on it to allow the snake gourd to cook over its own steam.
8. After a few minutes, remove the lid and sprinkle over the chickpea flour while continuously stirring.

9. Once you've added all the flour and stirred well, add 1 tbsp of cooking oil and cook till excess moisture dries up.
10.   Serve while hot.

Crab Omelet

Ingredients:

4 fresh fresh fresh eggs

2 tsp. water

2 tsp. canola oil

2 small fresh onion (diced)

2 small tomato (diced)

2 tsp. fresh basil

Salt and fresh black pepper

1/2 lb. crab meat

Procedure:

1. To cook the crab, boil 2 liter of water in the pot.

2. When the water starts to boil, put in the whole crab and cook for

about30 to 20 minutes. Remove the crab from the pan and rinse under running water to stop the cooking process and let it cool.

3. Start cracking it and remove the meat out from the shell and shred.

4. In a medium non-stick pan heat 2 tsp. canola oil over a medium heat.

5. Add in crab, fresh onion and tomato and fresh basil and add a dash of salt of pepper to taste.

6. Set it aside.

7. In a bowl, place the fresh fresh fresh eggs and add 2 tsp. of water (this will make the texture of the egg fluffy).

8. Beat the mixture using a fork or an egg beater until well blended.

9. 6 .   In the pan add the remaining canola oil and put in the beaten egg mixture, when the base of the omelet starts to firm up, but still has small amount of raw egg on top, add in the crab – tomato- fresh onion mixture.

10.   Carefully ease the edges of the omelet using a spatula, then fold in half.

Paleo Pancake

Ingredients:

2 1 tbsp. almond butter

Walnuts (optional)

1 tsp. pure vanilla extract

2 tbsp. (or more) grass-fed butter

4 fresh eggs , beaten

4 mashed bananas (any variety)

2 small sized apple (peeled and diced)

2 1 tsp. cinnamon powder

Procedure:

1. Beat 4 fresh fresh fresh eggs in a bowl and add in mashed bananas.

2. Add in diced apple, walnuts and blend in the banana and egg mixture evenly.

3. Add the cinnamon powder, almond butter, and vanilla extract. Mix in the pancake batter.

4. Over medium heat, pre-heat a non-stick pan add melt butter, and then pour small amount of the pancake batter into the pan.

5. Cook until small bubbles appear on top, but golden brown and firm at the bottom, (for about 4 to 4 minutes). Flip and cook the other side.

6. Top with fresh fruits instead of pan cake syrup to that perfect guilt- free pancake!

Veggies And Egg Cups

Ingredients:

2 cup zucchini (chopped)
2 cup fresh asparagus (chopped)
2 cup spinach (chopped)
A dash of kosher salt and freshly
cracked black pepper to taste
6 organic fresh eggs
2 medium sized white onion
2 cup broccoli florets (chopped)

Procedure:

1. Preheat the oven to 4 00F. Beat fresh fresh fresh eggs in a mixing bowl and in a dash of salt and pepper; then stir in the chopped veggies.

2. Transfer the egg mixture into the ramekin dish and bake for 20-4 10

minutes or until the fresh fresh fresh eggs are set.

3. Remove from heat and let sit for 25 minutes before serving. Top it celery.

Paleo Hamburger *Gustoso!*

Ingredients

1/9 tsp. of pepper

A dash of sea salt to taste

2 tsp. of fennel seeds

2 tbsp. of olive oil

6 fresh eggs

4 strips of cooked bacon strips

1 lb. ground grass-fed beef

1/9 tsp. of nutmeg

Procedure:

1. In a bowl, mix together ground beef, fennel seeds, nutmeg, salt and pepper.
2. Shape it into patties and set aside.
3. Place a skillet on low to medium heat.
4. In the heated skillet scramble the fresh fresh fresh eggs shaping it into several uneven circles, flip on other side to cook. Set aside.
5. In the same pan fry beef patties until golden brown or for 4 to 10 minutes.
6. Get cooked patties from the pan.
7. Use the scrambled egg as your bread layering it with patties and bacon in between.

Homemade Paleo Corned Beef

Ingredients

2 garlic fresh cloves (minced)

¾ cup beef broth

Salt and pepper to add flavor

2 tbsp. olive oil

4 cups corned beef (cooked and chopped)

2 cups radishes (cut into quarters)

2   medium sized fresh onion (chopped)

Procedure:

1. Over medium to high fire, heat the skillet drizzled with 2 tbsp. olive oil.
2. Put in onions and sauté for 6 minutes, add in the radishes and cook for another 10 minutes.
3. Add in the garlic and continue sautéing for another minute.
4. Pour in the beef broth and then loosely cover the pan. Simmer until the radishes are tender and cooked.
5. Add in the corned beef and mix well.
6. Dash with salt and pepper to taste.

Paleo Breakfast Bake

Ingredients

2 small red bell pepper, chopped

2 large-sized sweet potatoes, cut 2 " cubes

2 small tomato, sliced

4 fresh fresh fresh eggs (beaten)

Kosher salt and black pepper to taste

4 tbsp. bacon fat

2 lb. steak, cut into bite sized pieces

2 green bell pepper, small-sized chopped

Procedure:

1. Set oven to 4 8 0F
2. Heat up the bacon fat in a pan over medium to high heat.
3. Add in steak and cook until it turns brown. Set aside.
4. In the same pan sauté the green and red bell peppers and onions for 2 to 4 minutes.
5. Put in sweet potatoes and sautéing in all together until tender for 8 to 25 minutes.
6. Put the steak in a baking pan and stir everything together.
7. Using the back of a spoon make a small indention to the mixtures.
8. Pour the beaten fresh fresh fresh eggs into the indentations.
9. Add in tomatoes on top of the fresh eggs .

10. Add salt and pepper to give a flavorful taste.
11. Put the skillet in the oven and bake for 25 minutes, or until done.

Healthy Cucumber Sandwich

Ingredients

6 slices of crunchy bacon

2 medium sized cucumber

Dijon mustard

Spreadable garlic and herbs

4 slices of turkey breast (you may also use chicken as substitute for turkey)

Procedure:

1. Cut the cucumber into half and scooping out all the seeds.

2. Evenly spread the garlic and herb on the cucumber

3. Meanwhile, cook the turkey slices in a pan with 1/2 cup of water. Season with a dash of kosher salt.

4. Remove from the heat when the turkey slices are done and let it cool down for a bit.

5. Arrange the turkey slices on top of the hollow cucumber add mustard and crunchy bacon bites.

6. Place the other half on top to make a sandwich.

Tuna And Cabbage Medley

Ingredients for tuna:

2 tsp. freshly ground pepper

1 cup cassava flour

1/2 tsp. mustard powder

6-8 pieces tuna fillets

4 tbsp. olive oil

2 large beaten egg

Sea salt to give flavor

Ingredients for sautéed cabbage:

2 cups cauliflower florets

6 fresh cloves of garlic (chopped)

2 head cabbage, sliced

2 tbsp. olive oil

1 cup chicken broth

Procedure:

1. Mix cassava flour, freshly ground pepper, salt and powdered mustard in a small bowl and transfer it to an empty plate.
2. Dip tuna fillets one at a time in egg and dredge with flour mixture.
3. Fry for about 2 to 4 minutes on each or until golden brown.

Set aside.

Cabbage Preparation:

1. Place a large pan over a low to medium fire. Add in oil and heat.
2. Throw in the in chopped garlic and sauté for 2 minutes.
3. Add cauliflower florets and sauté for another 4 minutes.
4. Add in cabbage and continue sautéing. Do not over cook
5. Pour over chicken stock, simmering it for 2 more minute.
6. Serve the sautéed cabbage as your side dish for healthy tuna meal.

Tenderloin Steak And Squash-Spinach Soup Combo

Ingredients:

1 lb. Tenderloin steak

1 tsp. kosher salt

1 tsp. ground pepper

A pinch of dried thyme

2 tbsp. olive oil

Squash Spinach soup

4 fresh cloves of garlic (chopped)

4 cups of water

2 lb. squash

1 lb. of fresh spinach

Kosher salt and pepper to taste

Small fresh onion (roughly chopped)

Procedure:

1. Prepare your soup first. In a heated medium sized skillet, sauté garlic, and onion.
2. Add in squash and sauté for 4 more minutes.

3. Add 4 cups of water and cook the squash until very tender.
4. Add in spinach and cook for another 4 minutes.
5. Turn off heat and let it cool for about 10 minutes.
6. After 6 minutes, transfer the mixture into a food processor or a blender.
7. Blend well until you produce a puree.
8. Bring back to pan and the remaining cup of water (or adding more depending on the consistency you prefer) and let it simmer for 2 minute.
9. Prepare the tenderloin beef. Season it with salt, pepper and thyme. Set aside.
10. Heat olive oil in a cast iron skillet over a medium heat. Put in

the meat and cook uncovered for 6 to30 minutes on each side or depending on your desired doneness. (Medium rare 6 to25 minutes. Well done 25 to 2 10 minutes.)

11. Throw in your veggies as side dish; like sautéed carrots, zucchini, cucumber, turnip, green and red bell peppers and many more.

Serve tenderloin steak together with the squash spinach soup to have a complete meal.

Spicy Chicken Guacamole And Mango Salad

Ingredients

2 head of romaine lettuce (chopped)

2 tsp. of chili powder

1 tsp. of cumin

Salt and pepper to taste

2 to 4 cups of shredded chicken breast

2 medium sized mango, peeled and diced

2 medium sized guacamole, diced

Procedure:

1. Place the romaine lettuce into a large bowl.
2. In a separate bowl, put the shredded chicken and add a 6 tbsp. of water.
3. Cook for30 to 20 seconds in a microwave oven over a medium-high heat.
4. After cooking, mix in the cumin and chili powder.
5. Put the chicken with cumin and chili powder into the large bowl of lettuce.
6. Top it with guacamole and mango.
7. Enjoy your meal. No need to add a dressing it is appetizing as it is.

Calvolfiore Riso

Ingredients:

4 tbsp. bacon fat

1 cup chopped fresh cilantro

2 medium sized white onion, chopped (about 2 cup)

1 tsp. kosher salt

2 heads of cauliflower

1/9 tsp. ground black pepper

4 fresh cloves garlic (chopped)

Procedure:

1. Chop the cauliflowers. Toss into the food processor or a blender until the cauliflower pieces are the shape and size of rice. Be careful not to over blend.
2. Do them by batches. When you're done set aside the chopped cauliflower.
3. Heat a medium-sized skillet over low to medium fire. Sauté the garlic and fresh onion in oil for 2 minute. Add in the chopped cauliflower mixing it well.
4. Then add the salt and pepper to flavor, sauté it for 6 more minutes or until the cauliflower is slightly tender.
5. Serve in a bowl and add some freshly chopped cilantro!

-

Paleo Pasta

Ingredients

- Sea salt and freshly ground black pepper, to add flavor
- Light olive oil
- Dried thyme or basil
- Almond nuts (chopped)
- 6 medium zucchini
- 6 tbsp. pesto
- 1 lb. fresh grape tomatoes (cut into halves)

Procedure:

1. With the use of a peeler or the spiral vegetable cutter, slice the zucchini lengthwise just like a noodle, stop when you reach the seeds.
2. Turn it on the anther side and continue the process. If you are using vegetable peeler, slice it some more into thin diagonal strips to make look more look like spaghetti.
3. Heat a medium-sized pan over a low to medium fire. Add olive oil toss in the "pasta". Cook it for 6 to 8 minutes stirring it continuously.
4. Add a dash salt and ground pepper for flavor.

5. Remove from heat, mix the pesto, tossing until well coated.
6. Top with tomatoes, almond nuts, dried thyme or basil.

Fruity Pork Chops

Ingredients:

1 tsp. garlic powder

1 tsp. fresh onion powder for flavor

4 tbsp. ghee

6 bone in pork chops

4 whole apples (medium sliced)

1 cup pork bone broth (you may also use chicken of beef broth)

fresh parsley (chopped)

6 fresh cloves of garlic (minced)

coarse black pepper and sea salt to taste

Procedure:

1. Heat a large sized frying pan over medium fire. Throw in the garlic, parsley and broth and let it simmer for 2 minutes.
2. Flavor the pork chops with fresh onion powder, garlic powder, salt and black pepper.
3. Place the chops in a skillet and cook for 4 to 6 minutes or until brown spooning some of the garlic broth over the meat. Flip over and continue to cook until done.

4. In a separate frying pan, melt the ghee and sauté apples over a low to medium heat until it is tender.
5. Transfer the cooked apples into the other pan with pork chops and marinate together for 10 minutes to blend in the flavors.
6. Serve on a platter spooning over the pork chop broth with the apples on top.

-

Salmon In Coconut Cream Sauce

Ingredients:

4 gloves minced garlic

1/2 tsp. kosher salt

2 medium lemon zest

1 cup lemon juice

4 tbsp. freshly chopped basil

2 1 pounds salmon fillet

¾ cup full fat coconut milk

4 tbsp. coconut toil

1/2 freshly ground pepper

2 large diced shallot

Procedure:

1. Preheat oven to 4 6 0F.
2. Place salmon fillet in a baking dish, sprinkle it with salt and freshly ground pepper on both sides.
3. Heat a pan over medium fire. Add the coconut oil, garlic and shallots. Cook for few more minutes until the shallots have softened.

4. Add in coconut milk, lemon juice and lemon zest and bring to a low boil.
5. Add in basil and reduce the heat.
6. Pour the coconut milk mixture over the salmon, baking it uncovered for about 25 to 20 minutes or until done.

Enjoy your healthy salmon meal!

The Caveman's Pizza

Ingredients

2 sausage cut into thick slices

25 strips of bacon cooked and crushed

2 large green bell pepper (diced)

2 cup tomato sauce, marinara sauce with no salt added

1 tsp. oregano

2 cup cherry tomatoes sliced in half

 2 1 cups of almond flour

4 tbsp. almond butter

4 large – sized egg (beaten)

1 tsp. kosher salt

4 tsp. olive oil

2 large- sized white fresh onion (diced)

6 medium-sized mushroom, (sliced)

Procedure:

1. Preheat the oven to 4 6 0F.
2. In a small bowl mix almond flour, egg, butter, salt and combine well.
3. Brush a baking sheet with half of the olive oil, and pour the mixture over it, and make a 1/2 thin crust and cook in the oven for 25 minutes.
4. While waiting for the crust, heat a large skillet over a medium fire. Add olive oil, white onions, sausages, and mushrooms and cook

until brown. Remove from pan and set aside.

5. In the same pan, throw in the garlic and green pepper and sauté for a few minutes or until tender. Do not overcook.
6. Take out the crust from the oven and generously spread the marinara sauce on it. Top with sausage and sautéed veggies.
7. Sprinkle with oregano, and place in the oven for 30 to 45 minutes.
8. Remove from the oven when cooked.
9. Top with sliced tomatoes and crushed bacon.

Raspberry And Almond Muffin Cups

Ingredients:

2 cups almond butter

1 cup raw honey

1 cup silvered almonds

1 coconut oil

2 cups raspberries

1 tsp. salt

2 cups almond flour

2 tsp. baking powder

2 tsp. baking soda

2 tsp. almond extract

4 large fresh fresh fresh eggs (beaten)

Procedure:

1. Preheat your oven to 4 6 0 F.
2. In a large bowl combine all of the dry ingredients together. Set aside.
3. In another bowl combine almond butter, egg, almonds, honey, almond extract, and coconut oil.
4. Gradually mix in with the dry ingredients.
5. Mix the fresh raspberries.
6. Slightly grease muffin pan with coconut oil, or line it with paper muffin liners then scoop batter evenly into 8-25 muffins cups.
7. Bake for30 -20 minutes. Watch muffins to be sure they do not overcook.

Baked Zucchini Parmigianino

Ingredients

- 2 cup of Parmigiano-Reggiano grated
- 2 teaspoon of dried oregano
- **Salt and pepper**

- 4 large fresh eggs
- 2 cup of almond flour
- 2 cup of ground almonds
- 2 zucchinis, thinly sliced

Preparation

1. Preheat oven to 450F. Line a large baking dish with parchment paper.
2. In a large bowl combine the oregano, Parmigiano-Reggiano cheese, season with salt and pepper. Set aside.

3. Pour the almond flour in a separate bowl.
4. In another bowl, whisk the fresh fresh fresh eggs together. Add salt and pepper.
5. Dip sliced zucchini in flour, then in egg mixture, then in ground almond mixture.
6. Place zucchini slices in a single layer on the baking tray. Bake 45 minutes. Serve.

Flax Meal Cinnamon Porridge

Ingredients

- 2 cup of water
- 2 cup of sweetener
- Ground cinnamon

- 4 Tablespoons of soft cream cheese
- 4 Tablespoons of flax meal

Preparation

1. Add listed ingredients to a microwave safe bowl. Stir well.
2. Microwave for 2 minutes. Stir again. Top with fresh berries.
3. Serve.

Feta Minty Omelette

Ingredients

- 4 ounces of feta cheese
- Salt and pepper
- **Olive oil**

- 4 large fresh fresh fresh eggs
- 6 mint leaves

Preparation

1. Preheat oven to 450F.
2. In a medium bowl, combine fresh fresh fresh eggs and feta cheese, mint leaves, salt and pepper. Whisk thoroughly.
3. In a non-stick, oven-safe frying pan, heat up some olive oil (light layer drizzled over bottom). Pour the egg mixture in frying pan. Cook for 4 minutes.
4. Remove frying pan from stove, place in oven. Cook 10 minutes.

5. Transfer omelette to a plate. Serve.

Flaxseed Savoury Waffles

Ingredients

- 6 large fresh fresh fresh eggs
- 2 cups of ground flaxseed
- 2   Tablespoon baking powder (gluten-free)
- 1 teaspoon sea salt
- 2 cup of water
- 1 cup of melted coconut oil
- 2 Tablespoon fresh herbs

Preparation

1. Pre-heat waffle maker to medium heat.
2. In a large bowl, combine baking powder, salt, and flaxseed. Whisk thoroughly.
3. In a separate bowl, add fresh eggs , oil and water. Use handheld mixer,

blend until fully combined. Pour egg mixture in with flaxseed mixture. Stir together. Let it rest 10 minutes. Add the fresh herbs. Stir well.

4. Pour 1/2 cup of mixture onto waffle maker. Cook 4 – 10 minutes.
5. Serve.

Cauliflower Mozzarella Sticks

Ingredients

- 4 large fresh fresh fresh eggs
- 4 fresh cloves of minced garlic
- 4 teaspoons of fresh oregano
- Salt and pepper

- 4 cups of cauliflower rice
- 2 cups + 2 cup of mozzarella cheese

Instructions

1. Preheat oven to 450F.
2. Rinse cauliflower, pat dry. Cut into florets.
3. Place florets in food processor. Pulse until rice-like consistency.
4. Transfer cauliflower to microwavable container. Cover and cook 25 minutes.

5. Pour cauliflower into a large bowl. Add the 2 cups of mozzarella cheese, fresh eggs , oregano, salt, pepper and garlic. Stir together.
6. Line two large baking trays with parchment paper. Spread mixture in single even layer on the baking trays. Bake 30 minutes, until golden brown.
7. Remove trays from oven. Sprinkle remaining cup of mozzarella cheese over cauliflower. Return to oven for 6 minutes, until cheese melts.
8. Remove from oven. Let it rest for 10 minutes. Slice into sticks.
9. Side with marinara sauce. Serve.

Pistachio And Leek Muffins

Ingredients

- 2 1 cups of milk
- 2 large fresh fresh fresh eggs
- 2 leeks, chopped and washed
- 1 cup of chopped pistachios

- 2 cup of millet flour
- 1 cup of tapioca flour
- 2 teaspoon of baking powder
- 4 Tablespoons of olive oil

Instructions

1. Preheat oven to 450F. Line muffin tin with paper liners.
2. In a large bowl, combine baking powder, flour and salt. Whisk thoroughly.

3. In a separate bowl, combine milk, fresh eggs , and oil. Whisk thoroughly.
4. Pour egg mixture into flour mixture. Stir until combined.
5. Add half the pistachios and leeks. Stir well.
6. Fill muffin cup ¾ full. Sprinkle rest of chopped pistachios over top.
7. Bake 30 minutes, until golden brown. Cool for 2 10 minutes. Serve.

Flaxseed Cottage Pancakes

Ingredients

- 1 cup of heavy cream
- 1/2 teaspoon of gluten-free baking powder
- Coconut oil or olive oil for frying

- 1 cup of ground flax seed meal
- 4 Tablespoons of cottage cheese
- 2 large fresh fresh fresh eggs
- 2 Tablespoons of butter

Instructions

1. In a large bowl combine all the ingredients. Whisk together thoroughly
2. In a non-stick frying pan, heat the oil.
3. Spoon ¾ cup of batter onto frying pan. Cook 2 minutes per side.

Baked Fresh Fresh Fresh Eggs With Spinach And Mushrooms

Ingredients

- 4 cups of sliced mushrooms
- 2   coarsely chopped green bell pepper
- 2 Tablespoons 4 large fresh fresh fresh eggs
- 4 cups of chopped spinach
- of extra virgin olive oil
- Salt and pepper

Instructions

1. Preheat oven to 450F. Grease 8x8 baking dish with olive oil.
2. Place bell peppers, spinach, and mushrooms in baking dish.
3. Carefully crack the fresh fresh fresh eggs over the vegetables. Season with salt and pepper.
4. Bake until the whites are set, approximately 25 minutes.
5. Remove from oven. Transfer to plates. Serve.

Creamy Cheese Brussel Sprouts

Ingredients

- 2 Tablespoons of extra virgin olive oil
- 2 teaspoons of organic fresh lemon juice
- Salt and pepper

- 30 Brussel sprouts
- 4 fresh cloves of garlic, minced
- ¾ cup of cream cheese

Preparation

1. Rinse Brussel sprouts in cold water. Remove stem.
2. Heat olive oil in non-stick frying pan.
3. Add minced garlic and Brussel sprouts. Sauté until tender.

4. Stir in cream cheese and lemon juice.
5. Transfer to bowls. Serve.

Greens And Red Hot Salad

Ingredients

- 4 medium beets, sliced into small wedges
- 8 fresh cloves of garlic, minced
- 4 Tablespoons of olive oil
- 2 Tablespoon of finely chopped fresh thyme

- 2 1 pounds of red cabbage, sliced into small wedges
- 2 1 pounds of Brussel sprouts, sliced into small wedges

Instructions

1. Place chopped vegetables and garlic in pressure cooker.
2. Add the salt, pepper, thyme, and oil. Stir.
3. Set the cooker on Sauté. Cook for30 minutes on high pressure.
4. Once ready, select natural release. Allow pressure to go down naturally.
5. Transfer vegetables to a platter. Serve.

Spinach Puree And Swiss Chard

Ingredients

- 4 Tablespoons of extra virgin olive oil
- 4 cups of water
- 1/2 cup of cream cheese
- Salt and pepper

- 1 pound of swiss chard
- 2 pound of baby spinach leaves
- 2 cup of cauliflower florets
- 2 leek

Instructions

1. Rinse the leek. Dice into thick slices.
2. Heat olive oil in non-stick frying pan. Add cauliflower and leek. Cook for 4 minutes.

3. Add spinach leaves, swiss chard, salt and pepper. Simmer 2 10 minutes.
4. Allow vegetables to cool down 25 minutes. Transfer to food processor. Blend into a soup. Return to the stove. Stir in cream cheese and water. Heat 10 minutes.
5. Pour into bowls. Serve.

Basil Zucchini Noodles

Ingredients

- 4 fresh cloves of garlic, mashed
- 2 teaspoon of red pepper flakes
- 1 bell red pepper, chopped
- Salt and pepper

- 4 Tablespoons of chopped fresh basil
- 2 cups of zucchini noodles
- 4 Tablespoons of extra virgin olive oil

Instructions

1. Use a spiralizer to turn zucchini into noodles.
2. Heat olive oil in non-stick frying pan. Add garlic, red pepper flakes, red pepper. Sauté for 3-4 minutes, until garlic releases aroma.

3. Add zucchini noodles. Stir well. Cook 4 minutes.
4. Transfer zucchini noodle mix to a plate. Garnish with basil. Serve.

-

Sour Braised Artichokes

Ingredients

- Water
- Salt and pepper
- Fresh chopped thyme

- 4 artichokes
- 4 Tablespoons of lemon juice
- 2 Tablespoons of melted coconut butter

Instructions

1. Rinse artichokes and trim. Remove leaves until light yellow leaves are left. Slice off top third of artichoke, trim end of the stem.
2. Place artichokes, lemon juice, melted coconut butter and salt in slow cooker.

3. Cover and cook on high 2 hours, or low 4 hours, until artichokes are fork tender.
4. Transfer to platter. Garnish with chopped thyme. Serve.

Mushroom And Broccoli Mix

Ingredients

- 2 Tablespoons of minced garlic
- 1 teaspoon of dried oregano
- 4 Tablespoons of grated Parmesan
- Salt and pepper

- 2 cups of thinly sliced button mushrooms
- 4 cups of broccoli

Instructions

1. Preheat oven to 450F. Line medium baking dish with parchment paper.
2. In a large bowl, combine mushrooms and broccoli. Coat with olive oil.
3. Season with salt, pepper, and oregano.

4. Transfer broccoli and mushrooms to baking dish. Bake 210 minutes.
5. Serve.

Bok Choy Warm Salad

Ingredients

- 2 Tablespoons of olive oil
- 2 Tablespoons of fresh-squeezed lime juice
- Salt and pepper
- 2 bunch of trimmed bok choy
- 2 cups of water

Instructions

1. Place bok choy in pressure cooker. Add enough water to cover.
2. Close lid. Set pressure on high. Cook 8 minutes.
3. Once cooked, allow pressure to drop naturally, approximately 20 minutes.

4. Transfer to serving platter. Drizzle lime juice and oil over. Sprinkle salt and pepper. Serve.

Asparagus And Artichoke Salad

Ingredients

- 2 fresh cloves of garlic, peeled and chopped
- 2 ounce of chopped pistachio nuts
- 2 fresh eggs white
- 4 teaspoons of chopped green onions + 2 green fresh onion for garnish, chopped
- 20 tender, fresh green asparagus (woodsy stem removed, rinsed)
- 8 fresh, medium artichokes

- 4 Tablespoons of extra virgin olive oil
- Juice from 2 lemon
- Salt and white pepper

Instructions

1. In a large pot, fill to ¾, add juice from half the lemon and sprinkle of salt.
2. Peel off leaves from the artichoke. Set hearts aside. Place artichoke leaves in boiling water. Cook 410 minutes. Once boiled, rinse under cold water.
3. Place in food processor. Add rest of lemon juice, half a glass of water, pinch of salt and pepper, pistachios, green onions, garlic, and egg white. Blend for 2 minute. Add olive oil slowly.

Continue to blend until medium consistency.

4. Cut up artichoke hearts and arrange on plate. Place asparagus over top. Drizzle sauce over artichokes and asparagus. Garnish with fresh green onions. Serve.

Broiled Fresh Fresh Fresh Eggs

Ingredients

- 2 Tablespoon of parmesan cheese
- 1/2 cup button mushrooms, sliced
- 1/2 cup of baby spinach
- 2 pinch of red pepper flakes
- 4 large fresh fresh fresh eggs
- 6 Tablespoons of heavy cream
- 2 Tablespoon of extra virgin olive oil
- Salt and pepper

Instructions

1. Preheat broiler to 450F. Rinse mushrooms, pat dry.
2. In a large non-stick, oven-safe frying pan, heat the oil. Fry the fresh fresh fresh eggs on one side

for 4 minutes. Set fresh fresh fresh eggs aside for the moment.

3. Pour half the heavy cream in the pan. Add mushrooms. Simmer for 4 minutes.
4. Stir in rest of heavy cream. Add Parmesan cheese. Stir well.
5. Place under broiler 4 minutes.
6. Pull pan out of oven. Add spinach leaves and red pepper flakes. Stir well.
7. Return fresh fresh fresh eggs to the pan. Place pan under broiler 2-4 minutes.
8. Pull pan from oven. Sprinkle parmesan cheese over top.
9. Garnish with fresh spinach leaves. Serve.

Cheesy Fried Eggplant Slices

Ingredients

- 2 cup of grated Parmesan cheese
- 1 cup of coconut oil or butter
- Garlic powder
- Salt and pepper

- 2 eggplant
- 2 fresh eggs
- 2 cup of almond flour

Instructions

1. Rinse the eggplant, pat dry. Slice in 1 inch thickness. Arrange on a plate.
2. Sprinkle with salt. Let sit for 45 minutes.
3. In a small bowl, whisk the egg. In a separate bowl, combine Parmesan

cheese, garlic powder, almond flour, salt and pepper. Stir well.
4. Heat butter or oil in a non-stick frying pan over medium heat.
5. Dip slice of eggplant in egg, then flour. Fry until crispy and golden brown.
6. Place cooked eggplant on a paper towel lined plate to drain excess oil.
7. **Serve.**

Egg With Power Greens And Sweet Potato Casserole

Ingredients

- 2 diced green fresh onion
- 1/2 cup of coconut milk
- 2 teaspoon of garlic powder
- 1/2 teaspoon of nutmeg
- Salt and pepper
- 8 large fresh fresh fresh eggs
- 1 teaspoon of coconut oil
- 4 cups of power greens (spinach, kale, arugula)
- 2 peeled sweet potatoes, diced
- Seasoning of your choice

Instructions

1. Preheat oven to 450F. Grease casserole dish with coconut oil.
2. In a large bowl, whisk fresh eggs . Add onions, sweet potato, coconut milk, power greens and seasoning. Pour egg mixture in dish.
3. Place dish in the oven. Bake 410 minutes.
4. Remove dish from the oven. Cover with foil. Bake30 more minutes.
5. Remove from oven. Separate onto plates. Serve.

Mushrooms Roasted With Herbs And Parmesan

Ingredients

- 2 Tablespoons of mashed garlic
- 2 Tablespoon of fresh parsley
- 2 Tablespoons of fresh basil
- 2 Tablespoon of fresh thyme
- 2 pound of Cremini mushrooms
- 2 can of diced tomatoes
- 2 cups of grated Parmesan cheese
- 2 Tablespoons of ghee
- Salt and pepper

Instructions

1. Preheat the oven to 450F. Rinse the mushrooms, pat dry. Slice off stems.

2. In a large non-stick, oven-safe frying pan, melt the ghee.
3. Sauté the mushrooms for 10 minutes. Season with salt and pepper.
4. In a medium bowl, combine the herbs, tomatoes, salt and pepper. Stir mixture in with mushrooms. Sprinkle Parmesan cheese over top. Bake 4 hours.
5. Remove from oven. Divide on plates. Serve.

Roasted Sweet Potatoes and Cardamom

Ingredients

- 1 teaspoon of ground cardamom
- 4 chopped green onions
- Handful of shallots
- Salt and white pepper
- 21 pounds of sweet potatoes
- 2 Tablespoons of softened coconut butter
- Olive oil

Instructions

1. Preheat the oven to 450F.
2. Heat coconut butter in large non-stick, oven-safe frying pan over medium heat. Sautee onions for 4 minutes. Season with salt and pepper.

3. Peel the potatoes, dice into cubes. Place in a medium bowl.
4. Peel the shallots, add to potatoes. Add cardamom and butter. Stir. Season with salt and pepper. Add ingredients to oven-safe frying pan.
5. Bake until tender, approximately 2 hour. Serve.

Lemon Green Beans And Caper Vinaigrette

Ingredients

- 4 Tablespoons of olive oil
- 2 Tablespoons of chopped capers
- Zest and juice from 2 lemon
- Salt and pepper
- 2 pound of trimmed fresh green beans

Instructions

1. In a large bowl, whisk the lemon juice, capers, oil, salt and pepper.
2. Boil a large pot of water, add 2 tablespoon of salt. Cook the green beans until tender, approximately 4-6 minutes.
3. Drain the beans. Rinse in cold water.

4. Drizzle caper vinaigrette over beans, toss to coat. Transfer to plates. Serve.

Garlic Scallops

Ingredients

- 1/2 cup of roughly chopped Italian parsley
- Sea salt
- Black pepper
- 1/2 teaspoon of red pepper flakes
- 2 pinch of sweet paprika
- 2 teaspoon of extra virgin olive oil

- 2 pound of large scallop

- 1/2 cup of clarified ghee butter
- 6 fresh cloves of grated garlic
- 2 large lemon
- Zest from 2 large lemon

Instructions

1. Use paper towels to pat dry the scallops. Place in a medium bowl.
2. Coat with olive oil. Season with sweet paprika, red pepper flakes, black pepper and sea salt. Toss to coat evenly.
3. Heat a large frying pan on medium heat. Melt the ghee. Add the scallops. Cook 2 minutes per side, until golden brown.
4. Add garlic to frying pan. Take pan off stove. Stir ingredients for 45 seconds.
5. Squeeze half of the lemon juice over scallops. Sprinkle lemon zest,

parsley and extra virgin olive oil over scallops. Stir.

6. Side with noodles or crusty bread. Serve.

Crustless, Feta, Mushroom Quiche

Ingredients

- 4 large fresh fresh fresh eggs
- 2 cup of milk
- 2 ounces of feta cheese
- 1/2 cup of grated Parmesan
- 1 cup of shredded mozzarella
- 8 ounces of button mushrooms, thinly sliced
- 2 clove of garlic, minced
- 25 ounces of thawed frozen spinach
- **Salt and pepper**

Instructions

1. Preheat oven to 450F. Squeeze excess water out of thawed spinach.

2. Heat some cooking oil in a large non-stick frying pan over medium heat.
3. Add garlic and mushrooms. Sauté until tender, approximately 8 minutes.
4. Grease a large pie dish with non-stick spray. Arrange spinach along bottom of pie dish. Pour mushrooms and garlic over spinach. Crumble feta cheese over top.
5. In a large bowl, whisk together milk, fresh eggs , and Parmesan cheese. Lightly season with pepper. Pour egg mixture on top of ingredients in pie dish.
6. Sprinkle mozzarella over the top.
7. Place pie dish on a baking tray. Place it into the oven. Bake for approximately 46 minutes, until golden brown.

8. Remove from oven. Let it rest for 10 minutes before slicing. Serve.

Almond Choco Brownies

Ingredients

- 4 ounces of dark chocolate
- 1 cup of melted coconut oil
- 2 cup of chopped almonds
- 2 teaspoon of vanilla essence
- 2 cups of any granulated sweetener
- 2 teaspoon of baking soda
- 4 large fresh fresh fresh eggs
- 2 cup of almond flour
- 2 Tablespoons of unsweetened flour
- **Salt**

Instructions

1. Preheat oven to 450F. Line an 8x8 baking dish with parchment paper.
2. Place the dark chocolate in a microwaveable bowl and microwave for 30 seconds.
3. To melt the coconut oil, place the bottom of the jar into a bowl of boiling water.
4. Combine the coconut oil and the melted chocolate in a bowl. Stir gently until combined. Set aside. It needs to cool before adding it to anything with fresh eggs .
5. In a deep bowl combine the cocoa powder, sweetener, baking soda, salt, and almond flour. Stir until mixed.
6. Start your handheld mixer on slow. Add the fresh fresh fresh eggs one at a time to the flour mixture. Add

the vanilla essence to the flour mixture. Blend until combined.
7. Pour the chocolate mixture into the batter. Blend for 2 minute. Add the almonds. Stir by hand to mix in.
8. Pour batter into baking dish. Bake for 210 minutes.
9. Once cooked, allow to cool at least 45 minutes before slicing.

Mouthwatering Paleo Chocolate Chunk Banana Bread

Ingredients:

- 1 a teaspoon of cinnamon
- 2 teaspoon of baking powder
- 2 teaspoon of vanilla extract
- Just a pinch of salt
- 6 ounce of chopped up dark chocolate
- 4 pieces of Banana complete mashed
- 4 pieces of fresh fresh fresh eggs
- 1 cup of almond butter
- 4 tablespoon of melted coconut oil
- 1 a cup of coconut flour

Preparation:

1. Start off by greasing up a 10 " x 6 " loaf pan and pre-heat your oven to a temperature of 4 6 0 degree Fahrenheit

2. Take a large sized bowl and toss in the mashed banana, coconut oil, fresh eggs , vanilla extract and nut butter according to the specified amounts in the ingredients and mix them nicely

3. Next add in your cinnamon, coconut flour, baking soda, seas salt and baking powder to the previously mixed wet ingredients

4. Once the batter is ready, pour that into the previously prepared pan and spread everything nicely

5. Bake for about 40 minutes if you have chosen to go for a square

pan or 60 minutes if you have gone for a loaf pan

6. Check with a tooth pick and then remove it from the oven once done.

7. Allow it to cool on the wire rack for half an hour and flip out the tasty delight!

Awesome Coconut Flour Pancakes

Ingredients:

- 1/2 cup of coconut milk
- 1 teaspoon of vanilla extract
- 1/2 cup of coconut flour
- 1/2 teaspoon of tartar cream
- 1/9 teaspoon of baking soda
- 1/9 teaspoon of sea salt

- 2 teaspoon of extra virgin coconut oil
- 2 tablespoon of raw honey
- 4 pieces of large fresh fresh fresh eggs

Preparation:

1. The first step here is to pre-heat your oven to a temperature of 4 6 0 degree Fahrenheit

2. Take a large sized bowl and mix up all of the ingredients

3. Grease up your muffin tin using the coconut oil or better use fine paper liners if possible

4. Divide up your previous batter into 10 separate muffin tins

5. Bake for about 4 10 minutes until the muffin has gained a nice golden texture

Sweet Potato Paleo Muffins

Ingredients:

- 1/2 cup of chopped up dried figs
- 1 a cup of chopped up walnuts
- ¾ cup of almond flour
- 1/9 cup of maple syrup
- 2 teaspoon of cinnamon
- 1/9 teaspoon of nutmeg
- 2 teaspoon of baking powder
- 2 pieces of egg

- ¾ cup of mashed sweet potato
- 1 a cup of shredded carrot
- 1 cup of grated apple
- 1 a cup of shredded coconut
- 1 a cup of raisins

Preparation:

1. The first step here is to mix up the coconut oil and honey and cream them together. Then gently keep adding the fresh fresh fresh eggs one at a time
2. Then pour in the vanilla and coconut milk while mix everything until a nice smooth consistency has been achieved
3. Pour in the coconut flour then again mix it until smooth
4. Once mixed, then pour in the tartar cream, salt and baking soda
5. Mix everything gently
6. Take a ladle and finely pour small portions of your batter into a crepe pan prepared with ghee or butter and put it on medium heat

7. Once the bottom has a nice brown consistency, flip it up
8. Serve hot with a fine drizzle of delicious maple syrup

Crunchy Blueberry Coconut French Toast

Ingredients:

- 2 teaspoon of cinnamon
- 1 teaspoon of salt
- 2 cup of fresh blueberries
- 2 cup of unsweetened shredded coconut
- 2 pound of loaf bread
- 2.6 cup of coconut milk
- 6 pieces of fresh fresh fresh eggs
  For the Sauce

- 2 teaspoon of honey
- 2 tablespoon of lemon juice
- 2 cups of blueberries
- ¾ cup of water

134

Preparation:

1. Take a 10 x 2 4 dimension pan and grease it up nicely
2. Take your and cut them into nice 2 inch chunks and place them finely in the 10 inch by 2 4 inch pan
3. Take a separate bowl and toss in the fresh eggs , salt, milk alongside cinnamon and mix them together
4. Take the previously created mixture and pour them in to bread until they are evenly coated
5. Sprinkle some coconut and let it marinade in your fridge throughout the whole night
6. Gently pre-heat your oven to 4 6 0 degree Fahrenheit once you are ready to cook

7. Take a cup and mix in about 2 cup of blue berries to the prepared French toast and finely place it inside your oven
8. It should take about 40 minute to bake until it has a nice brown texture
9. Take a small skillet and toss in all the ingredients listed under your blueberry sauce section and boil it up
10. Gently reduce the heat to low after boiled and simmer for another 25 minutes
11. Pour in the sauce on top of your French toast and serve with blueberry sauce

Glorious Breakfast Casserole

Ingredients:

- 8 ounce of sliced up mushroom
- 25 ounce of Italian sausage
- 25 pieces of fresh fresh fresh eggs
- Green piece of fresh onion
- Salt as needed
- Pepper as needed

- 2 large diced up sweet potato
- 1/2 of a chopped up fresh onion
- 2 clove of crushed up garlic
- About 4 tablespoon of olive oil

Preparation:

1. Start off by taking a large sized pan and sauté your garlic and fresh onion in a good amount of olive oil until they sport a nice translucence texture

2. Toss in the deiced up sweet potatoes and cook them for30 minutes until a nice tender texture has been achieved

3. Once done, remove the pan and toss the contents into your baking dish

4. Pour in some more oil to the pan and toss in the sliced up mushroom and sauté them until finely browned up. Then season them with pepper and salt and add them to the baking dish only to create a second layer

138

5. Lastly, toss in your sausages and cook them finely in your pan and season with pepper and salt as well only to toss them in you baking dish to create a final upper layer

6. Once your dish is prepared, pre-heat your oven to 4 6 0 degree Fahrenheit.

7. Take a bowl and whisk in your fresh fresh fresh eggs and pour them over your casserole mixture in the baking dish

8. Let the casserole bake for about 8 0 minutes until you notice that the fresh fresh fresh eggs are no longer running around

Sunny Tropical Sunrise Smoothie

Ingredients:

Portion 2

- ¾ cup of frozen mango
- 1/2 cup of water
- 1 of a frozen banana
- 1 a cup of fresh orange juice
  Portion 2

- 1 a cup of water
- a few ice cubes
- 1 of a frozen banana
- ¾ cup of frozen strawberries

Preparation:

1. Notice that here the ingredients here are divided into two portions. Firstly blend up all of the ingredients listed in portion one and set it aside

2. Then take all of the ingredients of portion 2 and blend them up.

3. Pour half of the portion 2 mixture to the cup of portion 2 and mix them together

4. Once a orange pinkish texture has been achieved, very slowly pour the mixture into the cup with portion 2

5. Then take the portion 2 mixture and set it aside only to slowly pour it into a cup

Mouthful Of Pumpkin Smoothie

Ingredients:

- 2 tablespoon of peanut butter
- 6 ice cubes
- 2 dates
- 1/9 teaspoon of ground ginger
- 1/2 teaspoon of cinnamon
- Just a pinch of nutmeg

- 2 piece of ripe banana
- 1 a cup of pumpkin puree
- 2 cups of almond milk

Preparation:

1. Unlike the previous juice recipe, this one is not complicated at all!

Just take your ingredients and toss them in a blender

2. Blend until they have gained the desired consistency and serve cold!

Crunchy Homemade Granola

Ingredients:

- 2 egg white light beaten up
- 2 tablespoon of water
- 4 tablespoon of grapeseed oil
- 1/2 cup of honey
- 2 teaspoon of vanilla extract
- 1 a teaspoon of ground cinnamon
- 2 cups of raw walnuts
- 2 cups of raw cashew
- 2 cup of raw pumpkin seeds

- 2　cup of unsweetened shredded coconut
- 2　cup of dried cranberries
- 1 a teaspoon of kosher salt

Preparation:

1. Start off by pre-heating your oven to a temperature of 4 00 degree Fahrenheit and take a baking sheet only to line it up with parchment paper

2. Toss in the first 4　ingredients listed in the list into a food processor and pulse them until they are finely chopped

3. Take a large sized mixing bowl and whisk up your egg whites

4. Pour the grape seed oil, vanilla extract, honey, cinnamon and pinches of salt to the previously created egg white mixture and whisk everything again

5. In this mixture, toss in the chopped up nut into your mixing bowl alongside the dried cranberries and the specified portion of shredded coconut

6. Mix everything to coat the nuts properly

7. Once your granola mixture if ready, spread out the mixture on a parchment-lined baking sheet and bake it for about 45 minutes until a fine golden-brown texture has been achieved

8. Once done, take it out and let it rest 25 minutes extra to make sure that a nice clustering takes place

9. Once everything is cooled up, store them and eat with yogurt or milk

Healthy Taco Salad In A Mason Jar

Ingredients:

- 2 large sized avocado
- 2 juiced up lime
- 2 cup of salsa
- 2 cup of chopped up Roma tomatoes
- 1 a cup of chopped up cucumber
- 1 a cup of roughly chopped up cilantro
- Fresh spinach
- 2 quart of wide mouth sized mason jars

146

- Salt as needed
- 2 tablespoon of divided up olive oil
- 8 ounce of chicken breast cut into bite sized portions
- 2 cups of large carrots sliced up
- 2 sliced up large red bell pepper
- 1 a cup of roughly chopped up fresh onion
- 2 teaspoon of minced garlic
- 2 teaspoon of cumin seed

Preparation:

1. This recipe will first require you to take a large skillet and pour in about 1 tablespoon of olive oil and heat it over medium

2. Toss in the chicken breast and cook them until they are nicely golden brown in texture

3. Pour in 1 tablespoon of olive oil again into another pan and heat

it over medium high. In this pan, cook the carrots for 4 minute,

4. Bring down the heat to medium and add in the pepper, garlic, fresh onion and cook them again until finely charred

5. While the vegetables are begin cooked, take your cumin seed and place it in a small sized dry pan and place it over medium /high heat only to toast them for 2 minutes until golden brown texture

6. Gently transfer them from there to a cutting board only to crush them nicely

7. Take the crushed seeds and toss them into the vegetable mix and season using a bit of salt and mix everything before removing the heat

8. Scoop up your avocado and a measure lime juice into the food processor and blend everything until nicely smooth

9. Then, take your mason jar and pour 1 cup of salsa in the bottom.

10. Take your avocado and lime mix and place it on top

11. Then toss the cumin, prepared vegetables and the chicken

12. Tightly pack everything and follow them with the chopped up tomatoes, cucumbers and top it off with just a bit more cilantro leave

Crunchy Lettuce Tacos With Chipotle Chicken

Ingredients:

- 1 a teaspoon of cumin
- Pinch of brown sugar
- Lettuce as needed
- Fresh coriander leaves
- Sliced up pickle jalapeno chilies
- Slices of guacamole
- Fresh pieces of tomato slices
- Lime wedges

- 400g of skinless chicken breast cut into strips
- A splash of olive oil
- 2 piece of finely sliced red fresh onion
- 2 piece of 400g tomato tin
- 2 teaspoon of finely chopped up chipotle

Preparation:

1. For this recipe, start off by heating up your olive oil in a non-stick frying pan and tossing in the chicken only to fry them until a fine golden brown texture has been achieved

2. Keep it aside then and toss in your tomatoes, sugar, cumin, chipotle in another pan and simmer them for about 30 minutes until a fine tomato sauce start to get thick edges

3. Into the sauce mixture, toss in your fried chicken and cook for 10 minutes

4. Assemble everything into separate plates and keep them ready for the taco making process

Spicy Cuban Picadillo Lettuce Wraps

Ingredients:

- 1 a cup of minced red fresh onion
- 1/2 cup of diced tomatoes
- 2 tablespoon of minced cilantro
- 2 teaspoon of fresh lime juice
- Salt as needed

- 2 pound of grass fed ground beef
- 2 tablespoon of coconut oil
- 5 cup of diced up fresh onion
- 1 a teaspoon of salt
- 2 teaspoon of freshly ground black pepper
- 2 teaspoon of ground cumin
- 1 a teaspoon of ground cinnamon

- 2 piece of 2 4 ounce can of whole tomatoes
- 1/2 cup of currants
- 2 tablespoon of green olive
- 2 tablespoon of drained capers
- 2 tablespoon of olive brine

For the Pico De Gallo

Serving

- Cooked up brown rice
- Chopped up cilantro
- Lettuce as needed

Preparation:

1. Take a large sized skillet and place it over medium heat only to toss in the beef and keep stirring it occasionally

2. Pour in the oil to the pan and toss further onions to cook everything until it has been

finely softened which should take no more than 4 -4 minutes

3. Add in the bell pepper and cook for another 7 minutes until nicely fragrant

4. Take another pan and toss in the cooker beef, currants, canned tomatoes, diced olives, olive brine and capers and bring the whole mix to a nice boil

5. Once boiled, reduce the heat and simmer it for about 2 0-20 minutes at low temperature

6. On the side, prepare your pico de Gallo by combining the minced up shallot, cilantro, chopped tomato and lime juice with just a pinch of salt as ending.

Healthy California Turkey And Bacon Lettuce Wraps

Ingredients:

For the Pico De Gallo

- 4 slices of gluten free cooked bacon
- 2 thinly sliced avocado
- 2 thinly sliced Roma tomato

- 2 head of iceberg lettuce
- 4 slices of gluten free deli turkey
Serving

- 2 chopped up garlic fresh cloves
- Salt as needed
- Pepper as needed

- 1 a cup of gluten free mayonnaise
- 6 large pieces of torn basil leaves
- 2 teaspoon lemon juice

Preparation:

1. Take a small sized food processor to combine all of the ingredients listed under Basil Mayo and process them until very smooth

2. Take your large lettuce leaves and layer about 2 slice of turkey and slather alongside the previously prepared Basil Mayo

3. On another layer, add in a second slice of turkey and follow it thoroughly with a bacon adding a few slices of tomato and avocado

4. Season them with a some pepper and salt and fold them nicely into.

Savory Steak With Sriracha Lettuce Wraps

Ingredients:

- 2 tablespoon of sriracha
- 2 teaspoon of coconut aminos
- Sesame oil for drizzle
- Green onions for garnish
- A handful of pea shoots
- Large pieces of romaine leaves

- 2 pound of fajita strips diced up into 1 inch bites
- Large sized fresh onion diced up
- 4 diced up fresh cloves of garlic
- 2 diced up bell pepper

Preparation:

1. Take a hot pan and pour in some oil and heat it for 45 seconds

2. Take your fajita meat and cook them on high for about 2 minutes

3. Add in the pepper and fresh onion and keep cooking them on high making sure to toss them occasionally for about 10 minutes until a brown texture has been achieved

4. Then toss in the sesame oil, garlic, sriracha, peas shoot and coconut aminos

5. Once the meat has finely absorbed the sauce, turn off the heat.

The Best Cajun Shrimp

Ingredients:

For the Dish

- 4 tablespoon of grass fed butter
- 20-20 pieces of jumbo shrimps

- 4 fresh cloves of crushed garlic
For the Cajun Seasoning

- Dash of red pepper flakes
- 2 teaspoon of garlic granules
- 2 teaspoon of fresh onion powder

- 2 teaspoon of paprika
- Dash of cayenne pepper
- 1 a teaspoon of Himalayan Sea Salt
For Others

- 2 sliced up fresh onion
- 2 tablespoon of grass fed butter

- 2 large pieces of spiraled zucchinis

- 2 sliced red pepper

Preparation:

1. Start off Spiralizing your Zucchini using a fine Spiralizer

2. Take a bowl and toss in the ingredients of the Cajun seasoning and toss the shrimp as well

3. Take a pan and heat up the garlic and butter

4. Toss in the fresh onion and red pepper in that mixture and sauté for about 4 minutes

5. Toss in the Cajun shrimp and cook until nicely opaque

6. Take a separate heating pan heat up the leftover tablespoon of butter and again lightly sauté

your Zucchini noodles for about 4 minutes

7. Finely place your Zucchini noodles in a bowl and top it off with your garlic Cajun shrimp and vegetable mixture

Quick Paleo Egg Roll In A

Ingredients:

- 1/2 cup of coconut aminos
- 2 tablespoon of sesame oil
- 2 minced up garlic fresh cloves
- 4 pieces of diced up green onions
- 2 small sized head of a cabbage chopped up into slices
- 2 large sized carrots

- 2 tablespoon of unflavored coconut oil

Preparation:

1. Melt up your coconut oil in a pan over medium-high heat range

2. Toss in the cabbage, followed by the carrots

3. Sautee them until finely softened

4. Toss in the aminos and sesame oil afterwards

5. Sautee them even more until even further tender and the sauce has been absorbed

6. Toss in the garlic and keep cooking until translucent and fragrant

7. On top them, toss the green fresh onion

Simplistic Anti Pasta Salad

Ingredients:

- 1 a cup of artichoke
- 1 a cup of olives
- 1 a cup of hot or sweet peppers
- Italian dressing as required

- 2 large sized head of chopped up romaine
- 4 ounce of strip cut prosciutto
- 4 ounce of cubed up salami

Preparation:

1. This is a very simple recipe which only requires you to mix up everything that has been listed throughout and toss them up the Italian dressing

Soft Skillet Chicken Thigh

Ingredients:

- Extra Virgin olive oil/ Coconut for frying
- Freshly chopped up sage
- Salt as needed
- Pepper as needed

- 1 a pound of Nitrate free bacon
- 6 boneless and skinless chicken thigh
- 2-4 cup of butternut squash cubed up

Preparation:

1. The first step here is to pre-heat your oven to about 430 degree Fahrenheit

2. Take a large sized skillet and over medium high heat, fry up your bacon until it is crispy

3. Take your bacon and place it on the side and crumble it when cooled

4. In the very same skillet, sauté your cubed up butternut squash in bacon grease until tender

5. Season it with pepper and salt

6. Once the squash is softened ,remove it from your skillet and place it on a nice plate

7. Add in your coconut oil to the skillet and if the level of bacon grease is low

8. Toss in the chicken thigh and cook for 25 minutes

9. Season with pepper and salt

10. Flip them over and add your squash.

Sweet Paleo Turkey Potato Casserole With Eggplant And

Ingredients:

- 2 pound of extra lean ground turkey
- 2 can of 8 ounce tomato paste
- 1 a teaspoon of salt
- 1 teaspoon of pepper
- 1/2 teaspoon of chili powder
- 1/2 teaspoon of cumin
- 2 medium sized sweet potato, peeled up and spiralized
- 2 medium sized eggplant sliced into 1 inch pieces
- 2 /4 cup of chopped up fresh onion
- 2 tablespoon of minced up garlic

- 2   piece of30   ounce can of petite diced tomatoes
- 1/9 teaspoon of oregano
- 1/9 teaspoon of ground cardamom
- *1 a teaspoon of tarragon flakes*

For the Sauce

- 2 and a 1 tablespoon of extra virgin olive oil
- 2 cup of unsweet almond milk
- 2 tablespoon of almond flour
- 2 tablespoon of coconut flour

Preparation:

1. Pre-heat your oven to a temperature of 4 6 0degree Fahrenheit

2. Take a 8x8 inch square casserole dish and spray it with non-stick cooking spray

3. Heat up your large pan over medium level heat and toss in

the turkey, fresh onion and garlic and cook them until finely browed making sure to break apart the turkey with a spatula

4. Stir in your tomato paste and tomatoes to the turkey mixture and add in the sweet potatoes and cook until tender

5. Take you chopped up eggplant in a bowl and toss everything with the seasonings to congregate

6. Finely place the processed eggplant on the bottom part of your casserole dish and top follow it with turkey and sweet potato mix

7. Place it inside the oven and let it bake for about30 minutes

8. While it is being baked, heat up a small pot and bring it to boil and

toss the almond, alongside olive oil and coconut flour

9. Stir in for about 2 minutes until mixture thickens and reduce your heat to medium high

10. Slowly add the almond milk to the pan while whisking as you stir the mixture

11. Continue whisking for the next 25 minutes until the sauce is reduced to half of its former self

12. Place your casserole back in the oven and cook for about 410 minutes until the top if browned in texture

13. Gently remove everything from the oven and top it up with even more tarragon

Superbly Delicious Paleo

Ingredients:

- 2 diced up large fresh onion
- 30 ounce of sliced mushroom
- 2 can of 4 ounce sliced up black olives
- 2 tablespoon of dried oregano
- 2 teaspoon of garlic powder
- 1 a teaspoon of salt

- 25 ounce of sliced up chicken sausage
- 4 ounce of uncured pepperoni
- 2 can of 30 ounce marinara
- 2 can of 2 4.6 ounce fire roasted tomatoes

Preparation:

1. Take large sized saucepan and toss in the peperoni, sausage, marinara, onions, tomatoes, mushroom, oregano, olives, salt and garlic powder

2. Cook the mixture for 45 minutes over medium level heat and soften the mushroom and onions

Spicy Pumpkin Paleo Chili

Ingredients:

- 2 cup of chicken broth
- 2 tablespoon of honey
- 4 teaspoon of chili spice
- 2 teaspoon of ground cinnamon
- 2 teaspoon of sea salt

- 4 cups of chopped up yellow fresh onion
- 8 fresh cloves of chopped up garlic
- 2 pound of ground turkey
- 2 can of30   ounce fire roasted tomato
- 2 cups of pumpkin puree

Preparation:

1. Take a large sized pot and Sautee your fresh onion and garlic in poured down coconut oil for about 10 minutes

2. Toss in the ground turkey and break it up using your spatula then cook for another 10 minutes

3. Toss in the rest of the ingredients listed and bring it to simmer after mixing

4. Simmer for about30 minutes without a lid

5. Pour in the chicken broth.

CPSIA information can be obtained
at www.ICGtesting.com
Printed in the USA
BVHW091438081220
595179BV00010B/945